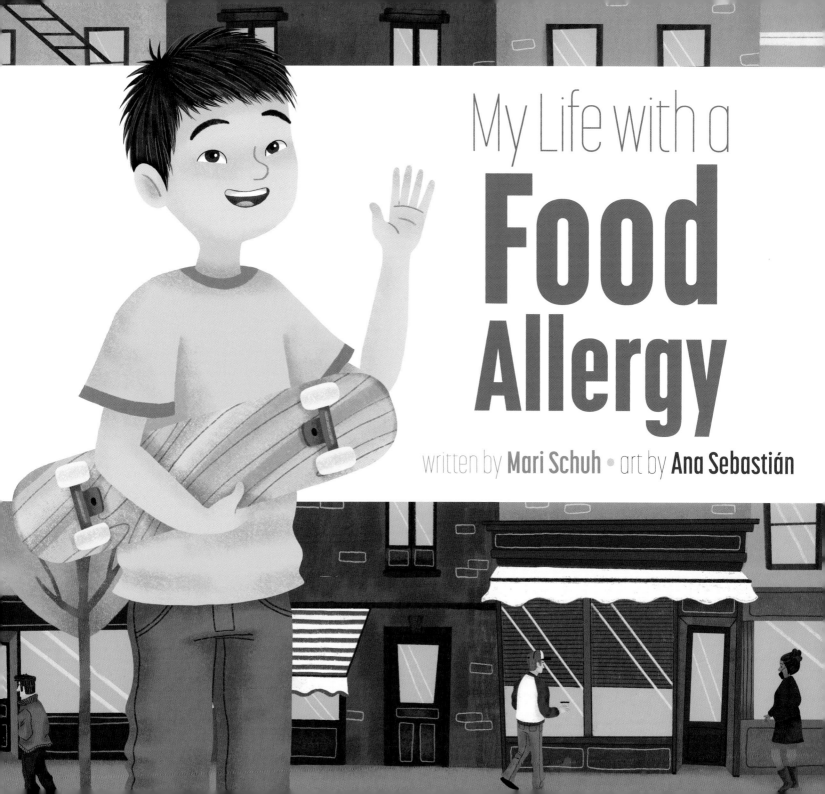

My Life with a
Food
Allergy

written by **Mari Schuh** • art by **Ana Sebastián**

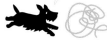

AMICUS ILLUSTRATED
is published by Amicus
P.O. Box 227, Mankato, MN 56002
www.amicuspublishing.us

Editor: Rebecca Glaser
Series Designer: Kathleen Petelinsek
Book Designer: Catherine Berthiaume

Library of Congress Cataloging-in-Publication Data
Names: Schuh, Mari C., 1975- author. | Sebastián, Ana, illustrator.
Title: My life with a food allergy / by Mari Schuh ; illustrated by Ana Sebastián.
Description: Mankato, Minnesota : Amicus Illustrated, [2023] | Series: My life with... | Includes bibliographical references. |
Audience: Ages 7 | Audience: Grades 2-3 | Summary: "Meet Hudson! He likes music and skateboarding. He also has a food allergy.
Hudson is real and so are his experiences. Learn about his life in this illustrated narrative
nonfiction picture book for elementary students."-- Provided by publisher.
Identifiers: LCCN 2021045835 (print) | LCCN 2021045836 (ebook) | ISBN 9781645494522 (hardcover) |
ISBN 9781681528595 (paperback) | ISBN 9781645494560 (adobe pdf)
Subjects: LCSH: Food allergy--Juvenile literature. | Food allergy in children--Juvenile literature.
Classification: LCC RC596 .S355 2023 (print) | LCC RC596 (ebook) | DDC 616.97/5--dc23
LC record available at https://lccn.loc.gov/2021045835
LC ebook record available at https://lccn.loc.gov/2021045836

For Hudson and his family–MS

About the Author

Mari Schuh's love of reading began with cereal boxes at the kitchen table. Today she is the author of hundreds of nonfiction books for beginning readers. With each book, Mari hopes she's helping kids learn a little bit more about the world around them. Find out more about her at marischuh.com.

About the Illustrator

Ana Sebastián is an illustrator living in Spain. She studied Fine Arts at University of Zaragoza and Université Michel de Montaigne, Bordeaux. Specializing in digital illustration she completed her education with a master's degree in digital illustration for concept art and visual development.

Hi! I'm Hudson. I bet we have a lot in common. I like music, baseball, and skateboarding. We might be different, too. I have a food allergy. Let me tell you a little about my life.

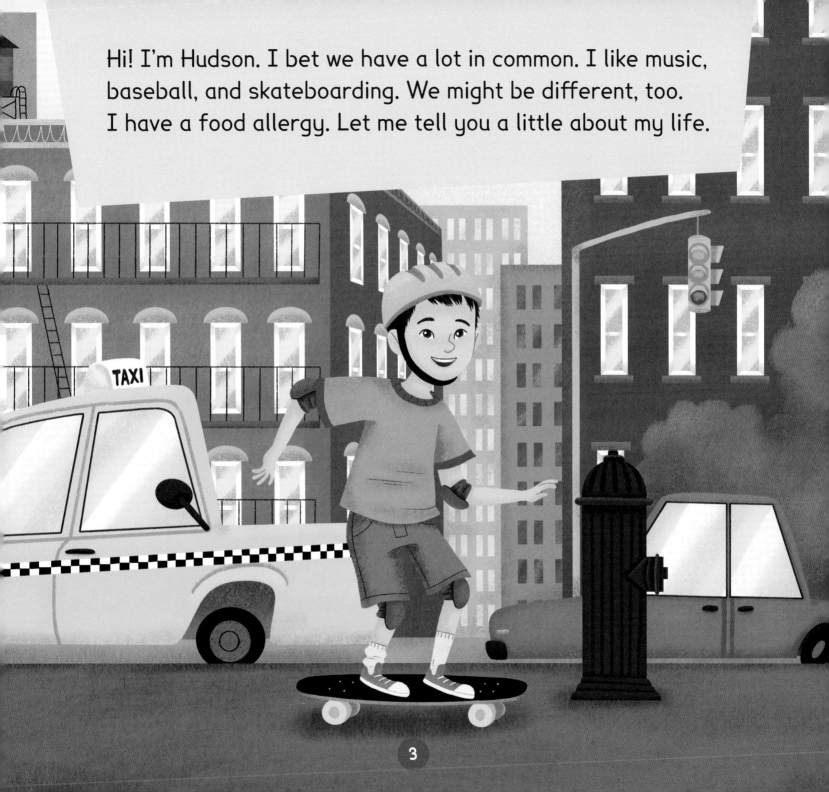

People like me who have food allergies can't eat certain foods. If we do, we could have a reaction, even from a tiny bit of food. Some reactions to food allergens are mild, like itching or hives. But others can be dangerous.

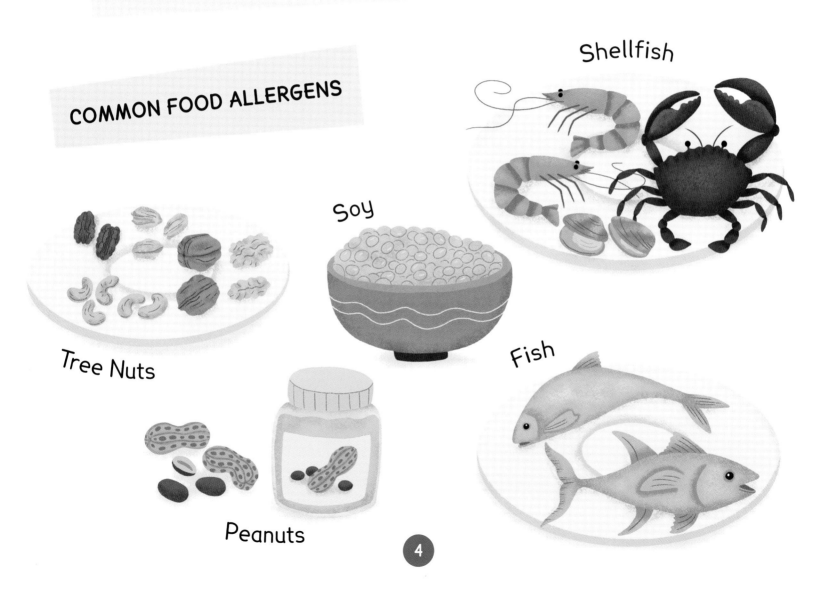

COMMON FOOD ALLERGENS

Shellfish

Soy

Tree Nuts

Fish

Peanuts

People can have trouble breathing. They might throw up, feel dizzy, or pass out. People carry allergy medicine with them to stop reactions quickly. It's shot into the leg with a pen-shaped dispenser.

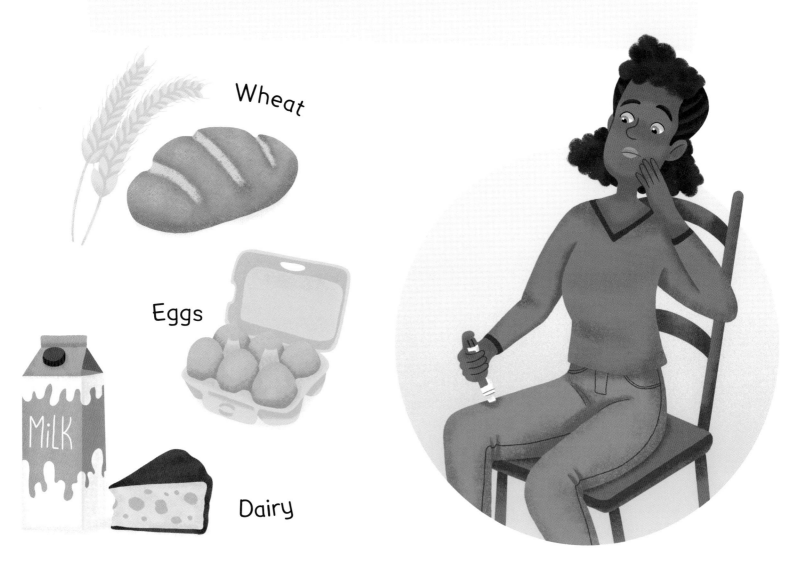

Wheat

Eggs

MiLK

Dairy

When I was very young, I ate some nuts as a snack one day. A rash formed around my mouth. That's when I found out I was allergic to tree nuts.

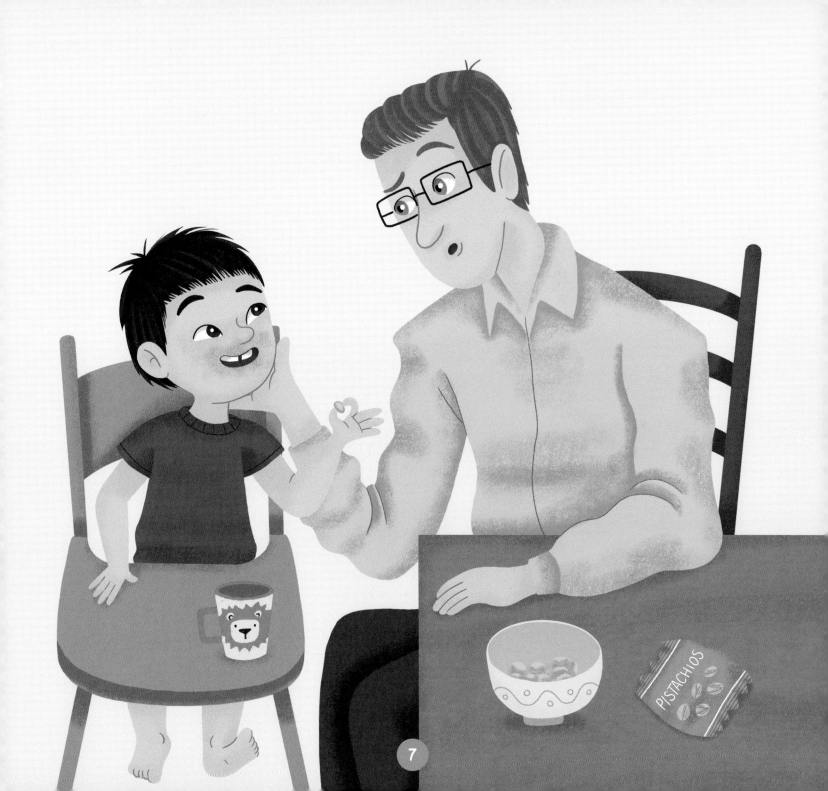

A few years later, I ate apple pie from a bakery. Grandma didn't know the pie had tree nuts in it. I coughed a lot and had a hard time breathing. An ambulance took me to the hospital. Doctors gave me medicine so I could breathe easier.

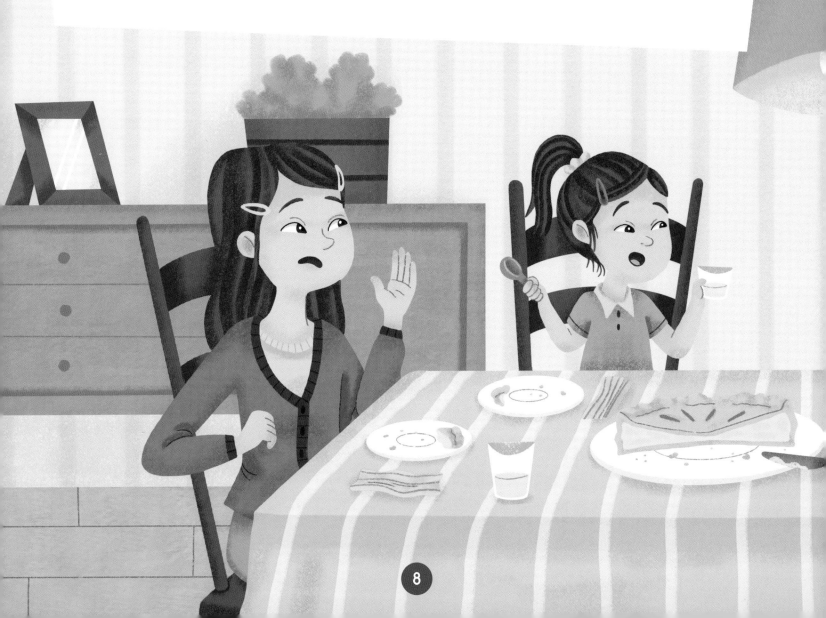

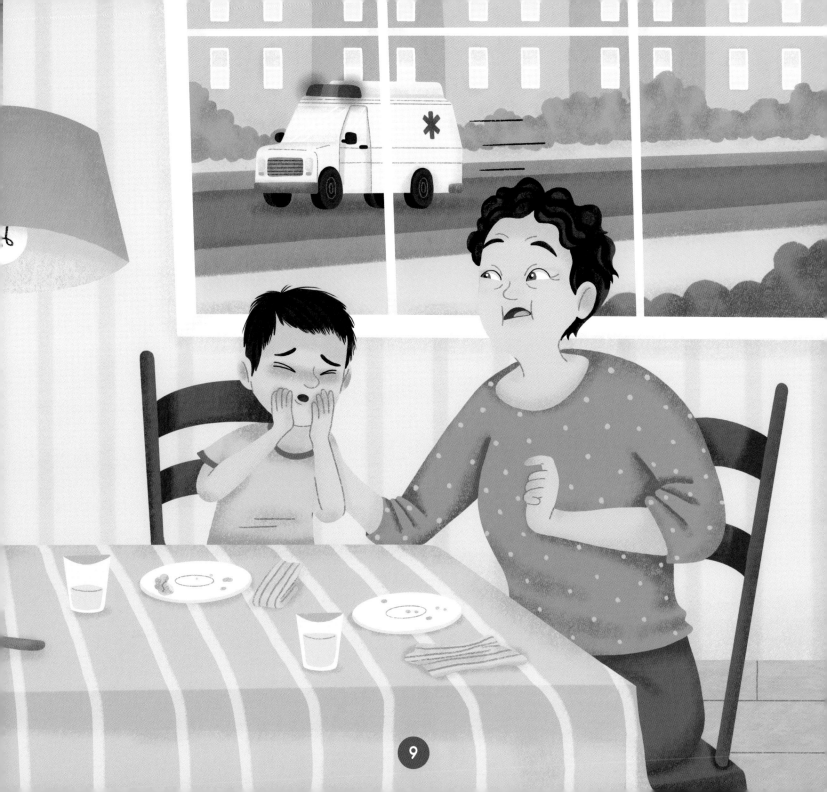

9

Now I'm very careful to avoid eating tree nuts. Sometimes it's hard to know if food has tree nuts in it. My family reads food labels all the time! Tree nuts are often in granola, cookies, cereal, and some breads. If I don't know if the food is safe for me, I don't eat it.

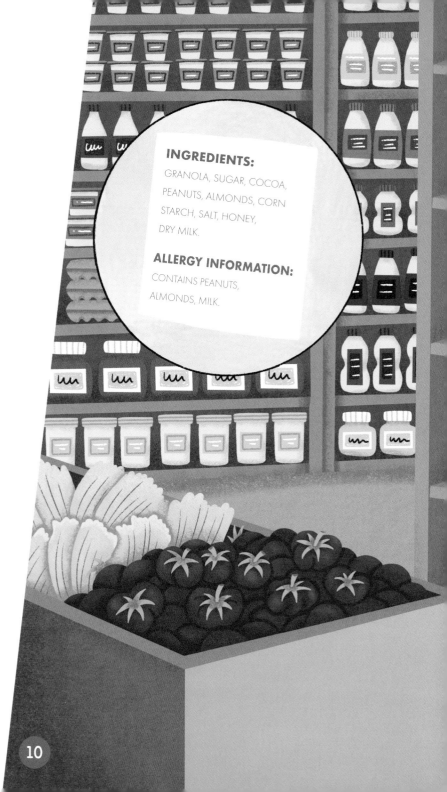

INGREDIENTS:
GRANOLA, SUGAR, COCOA, PEANUTS, ALMONDS, CORN STARCH, SALT, HONEY, DRY MILK.

ALLERGY INFORMATION:
CONTAINS PEANUTS, ALMONDS, MILK.

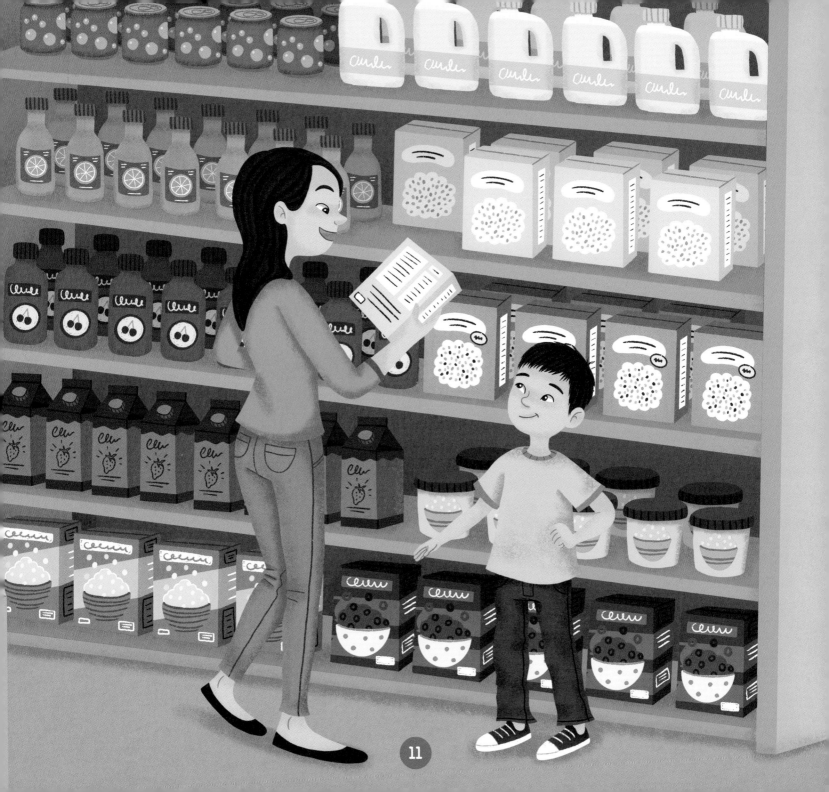

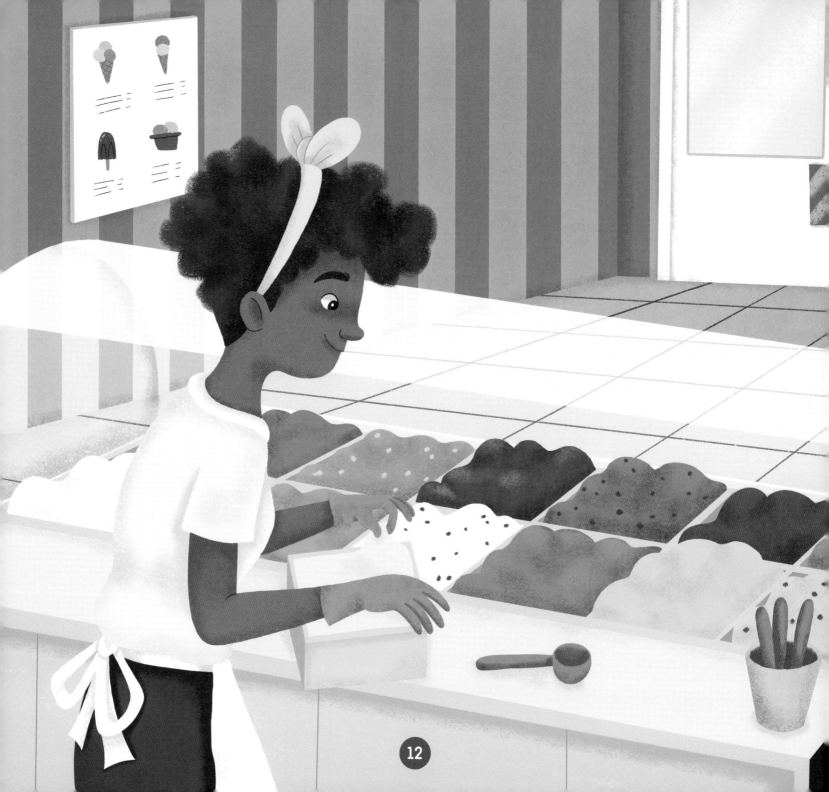

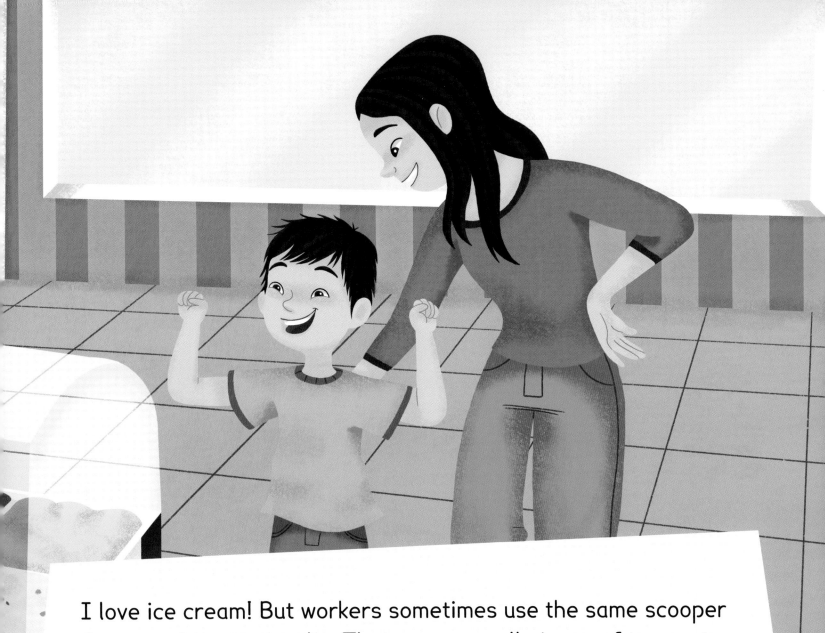

I love ice cream! But workers sometimes use the same scooper for many ice cream tubs. That means small pieces of tree nuts from one ice cream could get into another ice cream. So, I ask if they can open a new ice cream tub for me and use a new scooper.

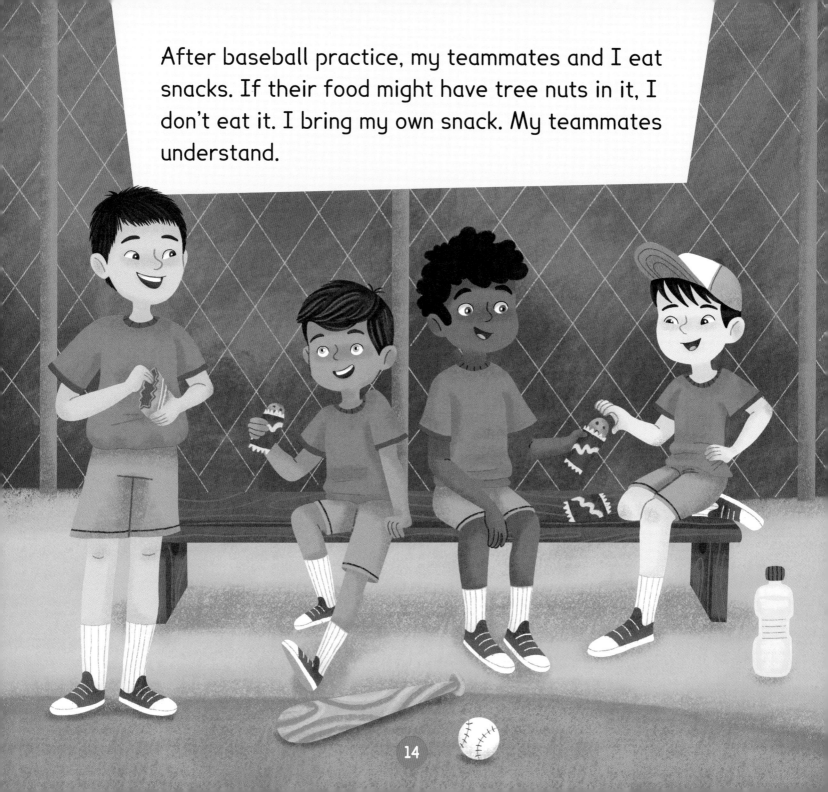

After baseball practice, my teammates and I eat snacks. If their food might have tree nuts in it, I don't eat it. I bring my own snack. My teammates understand.

Last week, I had a guitar recital. The teacher's wife made cookies for us. She made some cookies just for me! She made sure my cookies didn't have any tree nuts.

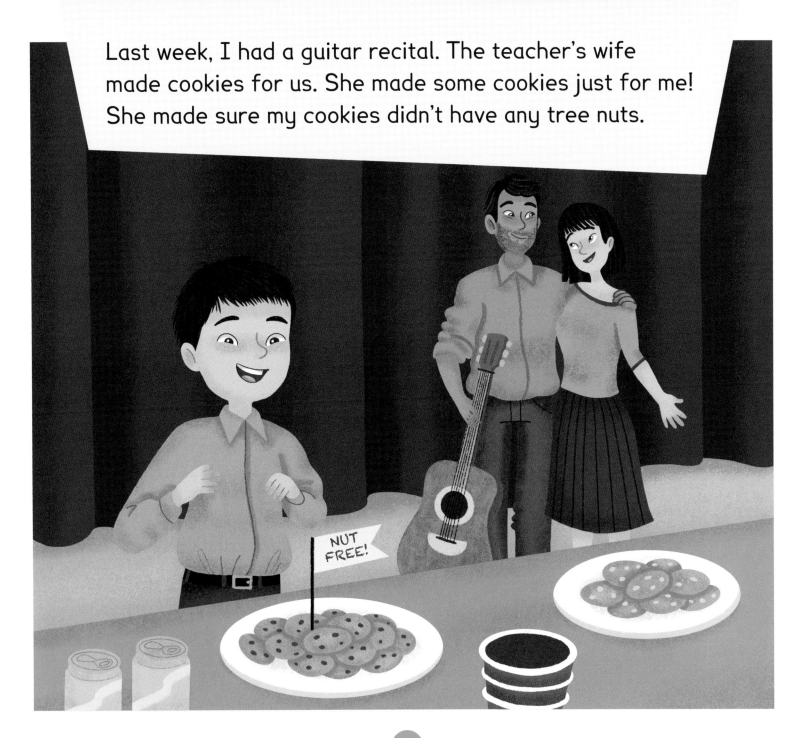

At school, I eat a sack lunch. Mom packs me safe, healthy food. My school helps me stay safe. Photos of kids with food allergies hang in the main office, so all the teachers know about them and can help us stay safe.

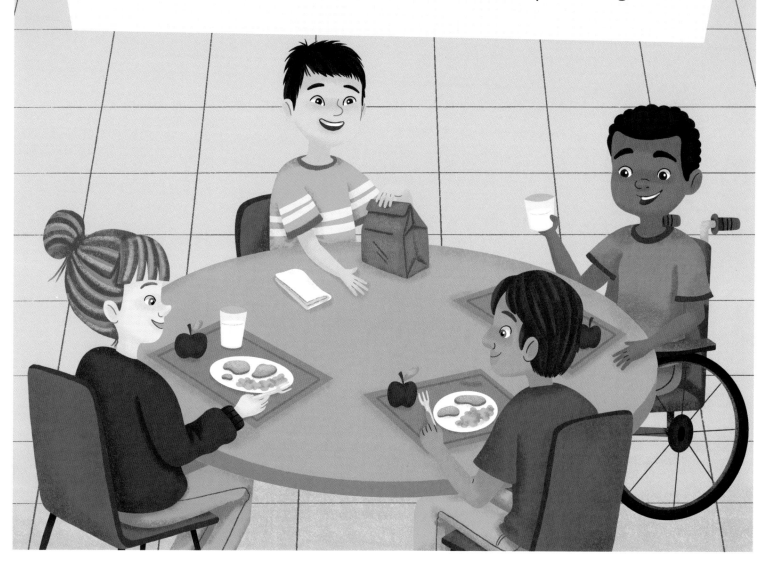

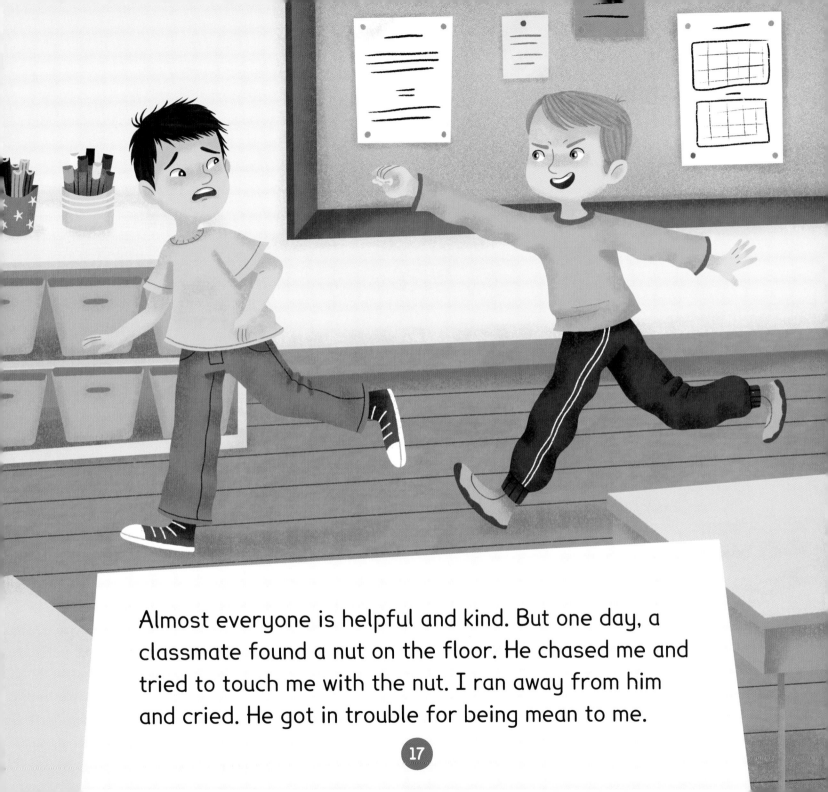

Almost everyone is helpful and kind. But one day, a classmate found a nut on the floor. He chased me and tried to touch me with the nut. I ran away from him and cried. He got in trouble for being mean to me.

Yesterday, our class had a birthday party. The birthday girl brought cupcakes for us. I couldn't eat them. No problem! My mom packed me my own treat.

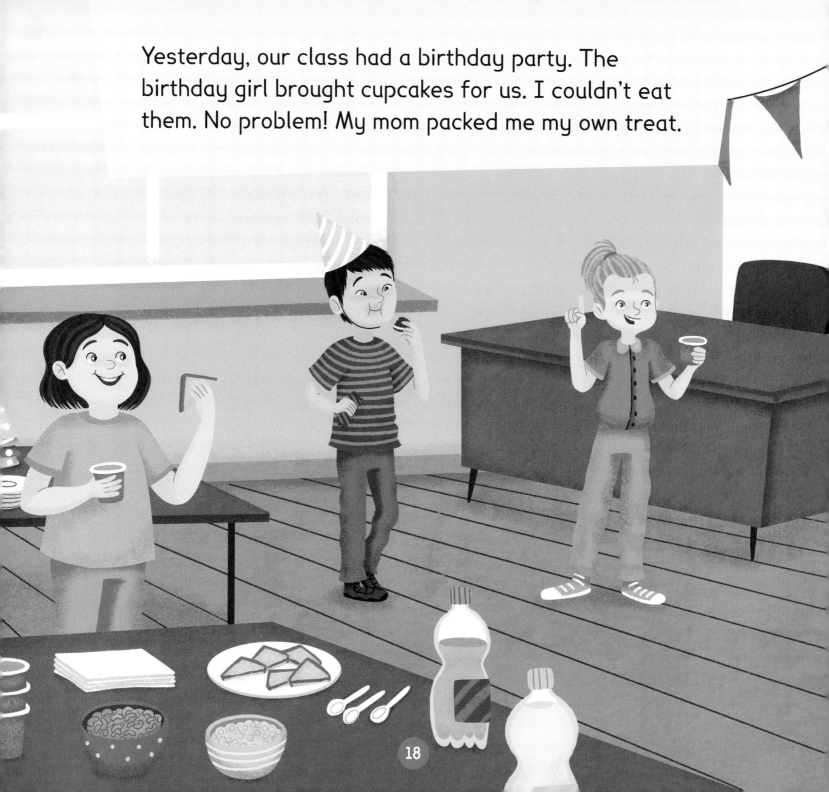

HAPPY BIRTHDAY !

Having a food allergy can be hard. I try to be positive. I focus on all the food I can eat instead of being sad about what I can't. This helps me see the good side of other things, too. Today it rained, and we couldn't go to the zoo. That's okay. My sisters and I stayed home and played games!

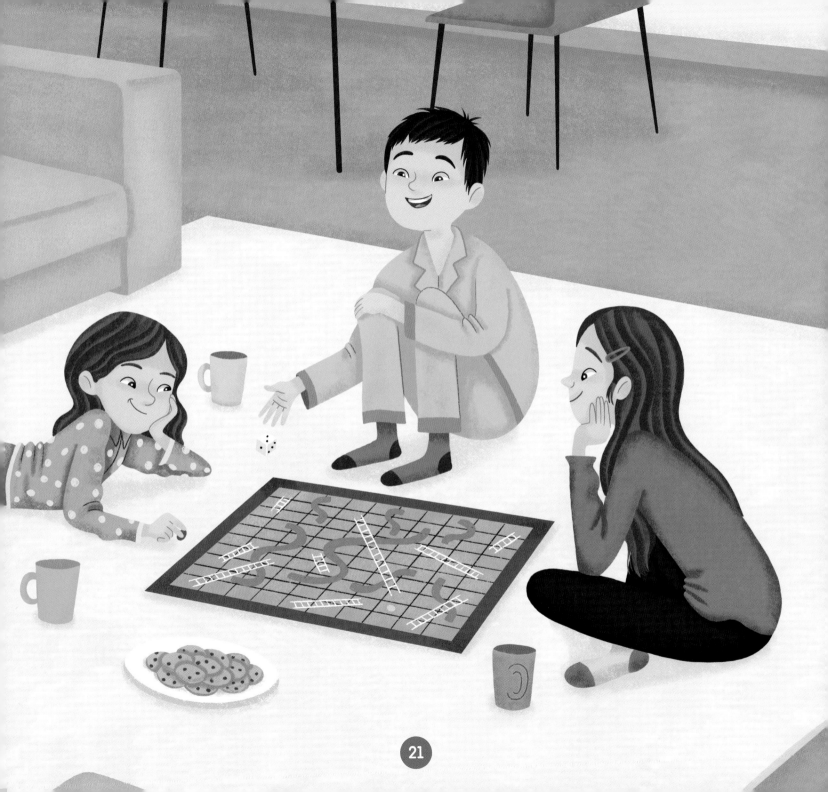

Meet Hudson

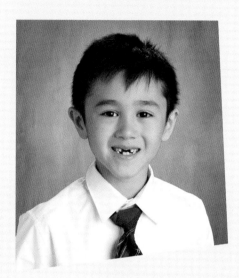

Hi! I am Hudson. I live in New York City with my mom, dad, and two sisters. When I'm not at school, I love to sing and play the guitar. I sing in the National Children's Choir. I also enjoy swimming, biking, and horseback riding. Some of my favorite foods are hash browns, pickles, and sushi.

Respecting People with Food Allergies

It's not easy to have a food allergy. Be kind and respectful if a friend can't eat what you eat. Don't make fun or tease.

Reading food labels takes time. Be patient. Remind them to check food labels if they forget.

If you see someone with food allergies having a reaction, tell an adult. Ask for help.

If a person with a food allergy can't eat the food you want to share, don't pressure them to eat it. They need to stay healthy and safe.

A person with a food allergy might feel different or embarrassed. Be a good friend to them.

When inviting people over to your house, ask your friends or their parents if anyone has food allergies. Try to serve foods your guests can eat. If you can't, ask them to bring their own food to enjoy.

Helpful Words

allergen   Something that causes an allergic reaction in some people.

allergy   A reaction in the body caused by something that is harmless for most people.

food label   An area on a food package that shows the nutrients and ingredients in the food. In the United States, food labels must list common allergens so people with allergies can avoid them.

hives   Raised bumps or welts, often red and itchy, that are caused by an allergic reaction.

rash   Red, itchy spots on the skin.

reaction   The body's response when it comes into contact with an allergen.

shellfish   An ocean animal with a hard outer covering. Clams, crabs, oysters, shrimp, and lobster are shellfish.

tree nuts   Nuts that grow on trees. Almonds, pecans, walnuts, cashews, and pistachios are types of tree nuts.

Read More

Corchin, D.J. **I Feel... Allergic**. Naperville: Sourcebooks eXplore, 2022.

Jorgensen, Katrina. **No Peanuts, No Problem!: Easy and Delicious Nut-Free Recipes for Kids with Allergies**. Allergy Aware Cookbooks. N. Mankato, Minn.: Capstone Press, 2017.

Kawa, Katie. **What Happens When Someone Has Allergies?** New York: KidHaven Publishing, 2020.

LaPlante, Walter. **I'm Allergic to Tree Nuts**. I'm Allergic. New York: Gareth Stevens Publishing, 2019.

Websites

KIDSHEALTH: FOOD ALLERGIES
https://kidshealth.org/en/kids/food-allergies.html
Read this website to learn more about food allergies.

PBS KIDS: ARTHUR FAMILY HEALTH: PEANUT ALLERGY
https://pbskids.org/arthur/health/allergy
Find helpful information about food allergies.

WONDEROPOLIS: WHY CAN'T SOME PEOPLE EAT PEANUTS?
https://www.wonderopolis.org/wonder/why-can-t-some-people-eat-peanuts
Learn more about food allergies from this education site.